MEDICAL PRACTICE MANAGEMENT
Body of Knowledge Review
Second Edition

VOLUME 7

Quality Management

Medical Group Management Association
102 Inverness Terrace East
Englewood, CO 80112-5306
877.275.6462
mgma.com

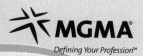

Defining Your Profession™

PRODUCTION CREDITS
Publisher: Marilee E. Aust
Composition: Glacier Publishing Services, Inc.
Cover Design: Ian Serff, Serff Creative Group, Inc.

LIBRARY OF CONGRESS CATALOGING-IN-PUBLICATION DATA

Quality management.
    p. ; cm. — (Medical practice management body of knowledge review (2nd ed.) ; v. 7)
   Includes bibliographical references and index.
   ISBN 978-1-56829-336-3
1. Medical offices—Management. 2. Medical care—Quality control. I. Medical Group Management Association. II. Series.
   [DNLM: 1. Quality Assurance, Health Care—organization & administration.
2. Practice Management—organization & administration. W 84.1 Q1546 2009]
   R728.Q35 2009
   610.68—dc22

                                                                    2008044482

Printed in the United States of America
10 9 8 7 6 5 4 3 2 1

Dedication

To our colleagues in the profession
of medical practice management
and to the groups that support us
in our efforts to serve our profession.

Body of Knowledge Review Series — Second Edition

Contents

Preface

TO SUCCEED AND FLOURISH in the day-to-day work environment of managing a medical practice, it is important that the successful administrator master and become adept at utilizing basic and advanced Quality Management skills.

The Quality Management domain within the *Medical Practice Management Body of Knowledge (BOK), second edition,* presents the basic building blocks needed to efficiently and effectively deliver high-quality health care and ensure patient safety of a medical group practice, regardless of its legal or political structure. Included within the general competency of critical thinking skills, the Quality Management domain requires an in-depth understanding of the other competencies (communication, professionalism, and skills) for the effective management of a group practice.

When faced with the task of assuming the leadership of a medical practice, the effective medical practice executive should properly utilize the basic tools of Quality Management and properly evaluate the issues affecting the organization. Through the proper application of these tools, the administrator will be able to prepare and implement the steps needed to place the organization on a firm footing for survival and growth. Examples of the organizational effects that result when these tools are put to proper use can be seen in many organizations and real life experiences.

Knowledge of the tools within the Quality Management domain and the way they interact with the other domains within the BOK affords the health care administrator the ability to provide the direction and leadership needed by his or her organization. These same tools are utilized in the day-to-day operation of a practice and assist the administrator in ensuring the continued growth and development of the organization.

Body of Knowledge Review Series Contributors

Geraldine Amori, PhD, ARM, CPHRM
Douglas G. Anderson, FACMPE
James A. Barnes, MBA
Fred Beck, JD
Jerry D. Callahan Jr., CPA
Anthony J. DiPiazza, CPA
David N. Gans, MSHA, FACMPE
Robert L. Garrie, MPA, RHIA
Edward Gulko, MBA, FACMPE, FACHE, LNHA
Kenneth T. Hertz, CMPE
Steven M. Hudson, CFP, CFS, CRPC
Jerry Lagle, MBA, CPA, FACMPE
Michael Landers
Gary Lewins, FACMPE, CPA, FHFMA
Ken Mace, MA, CMPE
Jeffrey Milburn, MBA, CMPE
Michael A. O'Connell, MHA, FACMPE, CHE
Dawn M. Oetjen, PhD, MHA
Reid M. Oetjen, PhD, MSHSA
Pamela E. Paustian, MSM, RHIA
David Peterson, MBA, FACMPE
Lisa H. Schneck, MSJ
Frederic R. Simmons Jr., CPA
Thomas E. Sisson, CPA
Donna J. Slovensky, PhD, RHIA, FAHIMA
Jerry M. Trimm, PhD, FHIMSS
Stephen L. Wagner, PhD, FACMPE
Lee Ann H. Webster, MA, CPA, FACMPE
Susan Wendling-Aloi, MPA, FACMPE
Warren C. White Jr., FACMPE
Lawrence Wolper, MBA, FACMPE, CMC
Lorraine C. Woods, FACMPE
James R. Wurts, FACMPE

Learning Objectives

AFTER READING THIS VOLUME, the medical practice executive will be able to accomplish the following tasks:

- Design and implement a quality management system that leads to the improvement of health care delivery and ensures patient safety;

- Develop and oversee patient satisfaction and customer service programs;

- Identify, develop, and maintain benchmarks for establishing practice performance standards;

- Create internal processes and systems to participate in pay-for-performance programs to enhance health care quality;

- Develop and monitor a program for staff, business, and equipment credentialing and licensure; and

- Monitor the peer review process for clinical staff.

Quality Quandary: Are You on Track to Establish a Medical Practice Quality Program?[1]

Third-party payers are initiating programs to pay medical practices for quality reporting. Many, including Medicare, have pilot programs in place with selected practices. Those initiatives are forming the basis for an industrywide shift to pay-for-performance systems, a response to consumer-driven health care.

Now is the time to initiate or improve your quality program. You should address five areas when your practice is ready to move forward:

- Organizational culture and support;
- Organizational systems readiness;
- Environmental changes;
- Partnering opportunities; and
- Steps to implementation.

This vignette provides ideas and resources to assist you with this process.

■ Organizational Culture and Support

The success of any program in your organization depends on leadership support. This is best developed through strategic planning that sets both short- and long-term goals. All practice leaders need to agree on the benefits of a quality program and on the steps to implement it. This can be accomplished by a SWOT (strengths, weaknesses, opportunities, and threats) analysis directed at a quality program.

If you and other leaders want to assess the practice before planning a quality program, the Malcolm Baldrige organization provides a free online assessment, specific to health care, at www.quality.nist .gov/eBaldrige/Step_One.htm. The assessment identifies areas needing work. The Baldrige Website has additional tools to apply structure to your work plan.

A key part of a quality program is setting compensation goals. This provides the financial incentive for support from physicians and staff. Most physician compensation plans are based on production. You can incorporate organizational goals into compensation plans with minor adjustments. Some medical groups also have incentive programs for staff, which help align employees' efforts with financial performance. Staff incentive programs can provide nonfinancial rewards or modest monetary compensation if financial goals are achieved.

■ Organizational Systems Readiness

Data capture and reporting compose a significant part of an effective quality program. An electronic health record (EHR) system can greatly simplify these efforts. However, a September 2005 survey of 3,300 medical practices found that only 14 percent had completed EHR implementation.[2]

Establishing such technology takes considerable time and effort. Groups need to consider this in setting quality indicators at the same time they implement an EHR. The system's design needs to incorporate quality reporting.

Consider your practice's coding program. An effective one offers:

- Periodic reporting of coding against industry benchmarks to all practitioners;
- Periodic audits with scoring of coding effectiveness; and
- The support of coding coaches for practitioners as questions arise.

If you don't have the major components of an effective coding program in place, you'll need to make those enhancements part of a systems readiness plan for quality reporting.

Help for Selecting an EHR

If your practice is considering an EHR system, industry assistance is available. Three leading health information-technology industry associations – the American Health Information Management Association, the Healthcare Information and Management Systems Society, and the National Alliance for Health Information Technology – joined forces to launch the Certification Commission for Healthcare Information Technology (CCHIT) as a voluntary, private-sector organization to certify health care information technology (www.cchit.org).

CCHIT provides a list of certified EHR vendors whose products have been extensively tested against a wide-ranging functionality and security criteria.

Outline of CMS Pay-for-Performance Program

The Tax Relief and Health Care Act of 2006 provides for a 1.5 percent bonus payment for Medicare data reporting. The Centers for Medicare and Medicaid Services (CMS) will use the taxpayer identification number to determine whether an individual physician or the medical practice will receive the payment in 2008. The agency has not yet determined the exact date of payment in 2008.

CMS has outlined 74 quality measures for 2007. To be eligible for the bonus, a provider must report at least 80 percent of the services for a particular measure. The information will become part of the 2007 Physician Quality Reporting Initiative (PQRI) database; eligible providers will have access to CMS analysis of their reported data in 2008. Detailed information about eligible health care professionals and the list of quality measures and reporting requirements can be found online at www.cms.hhs.gov/pqri.

Required reporting will be based on G codes or Current Procedural Terminology (CPT®) level II codes. The billing code reporting system is meant to be an interim reporting system. CMS plans to develop a system allowing medical practices to submit data directly from their practice EMR systems. Eligible professionals are encouraged to monitor www.qualitynet.org/ to find a model worksheet for data collection.

Commercial payers often follow Medicare's lead on payment systems. They have been developing quality information through the National Center for Quality Assurance (NCQA), which certifies managed care organizations. The NCQA has developed the Healthcare Effectiveness Data and Information Set (HEDIS), a set of standardized performance measures designed to ensure that purchasers and consumers have information to reliably compare the performance of managed health care plans.

HEDIS performance measures are related to many significant public health issues such as cancer, heart disease, smoking, asthma, and diabetes. HEDIS offers a standardized survey of consumers' experiences that evaluates plan performance in areas such as customer service, access to care, and claims processing.

The NCQA Website, www.ncqa.org, provides a table of the 2008 HEDIS measures, including a comparison of quality measures used by Medicare, Medicaid, and various commercial payers. The HEDIS measurement system includes elements of consumer satisfaction. It is important for medical practices to consider similar measures.

Partnering Opportunities

Implementing a quality program presents a significant challenge. You may find assistance from Medicare, local hospitals, medical specialty societies, and other medical practices.

The Medicare program has contracted with quality improvement organizations (QIOs) in each state to assist physician practices. Find contact information for each QIO at www.medqic.org. A number of QIOs have also contracted with peer-review groups throughout the country to provide quality reporting information. Those organizations can help medical groups establish a quality program and assist with the details of implementation.

Because hospitals have long been required to have quality programs in place to meet the requirements of the Joint Commission on Accreditation of Healthcare Organizations, they may be able to assist your practice in:

- Developing an implementation plan, based on hospital experience;

- Integrating quality information and reporting within an integrated delivery system; and

- Financing an EHR.

Medical practices that are a part of an integrated delivery system (IDS) will need to coordinate quality program development with other components of the IDS. Independent medical practices will need to develop separate quality reporting systems.

Recent rules from the Department of Health and Human Services created exceptions to the physician self-referral statute and a new safe harbor under the federal antikickback statute permitting hospitals and others to donate certain electronic prescribing and EHR technologies. Donations may make EHR systems more affordable for practices.

In addition, other medical practices further along in the process can help your organization. They can tell you the lessons they learned and advise you on steps to avoid.

▌ Steps to Implementation

An implementation plan for an effective quality program in your practice involves five key steps:

1. **Assessing your practice's readiness** – This includes the culture, leadership support, and compensation alignment. Organizational systems such as the EHR and an effective coding program must be incorporated into the implementation plan.

2. **Data gathering** – This includes knowing what payers in your area are doing and a decision about whether to participate in the PQRI to earn the 1.5 percent Medicare bonus payment. Gather other program information using the resources indicated.

3. **Setting the measures and reporting** – Ensure that systems are in place to gather accurate data and provide routine reporting.

4. **Identifying partners** – Use other potential partners to the fullest extent possible.

5. **Preparing an implementation plan and completing it** – The chance of success increases significantly with a well-developed and well-executed implementation plan.

Good luck with the new era of quality.

Current Quality Management Issues

WHEN LOOKING at the Quality Management domain from a broad perspective, it is clear that this domain is in a state of change. It is apparent that the domain is in a state of evolution as it attempts to maintain balance while also changing to meet the demands and expectations of the individual stakeholders as well as society as a whole. The practice administrator should take the time to identify and understand the specific pressures of achieving "quality" as well as those issues that are core within other domains but also affect this domain.

Numerous internal and external pressures affect the patient/clinical side of practice management. These pressures include, but are not limited to:

1. Monitoring the peer review and credentialing processes;

2. Implementing and reporting on patient satisfaction programs;

3. Choosing meaningful benchmarks to measure;

4. Creating processes to enhance health care quality; and

5. Constructing a data collection plan.

Knowledge Needs

TO PROPERLY AND EFFECTIVELY RESPOND to the ongoing internal and external forces on both the practice and business of medicine, the practice executive should be well grounded in the fundamentals of day-to-day operations and the methodologies needed to maintain and improve the processes that affect organizations during these ever-evolving times. Expertise in these fundamental Quality Management skills is the ultimate goal. Several of the key skills include the ability to use quality management tools and techniques to measure and improve practice operations; the development and implementation of survey and benchmarking techniques to identify expectations and perceived shortcomings among patients; and the identification of patient and organizational needs while evaluating, designing, and implementing changes to meet those needs. Finally, the medical practice executive needs to know how the various parts of the operation fit together and how they complement and support each other.

Quality Management includes six distinct tasks, as identified in this volume. Each task is interconnected with the others through two strong identifiable threads, namely:

1. Ensuring patient safety and satisfaction; and

2. Managing processes and programs for staff, business, and equipment credentialing and licensure.

Chapter 1 **Improving Health Care Delivery and Patient Safety**

◼ Process Improvement

Growth, change, and evolution constitute the goal and the reason to develop and implement process improvement programs within a practice. The practice that does not constantly test its own organization's core processes and develop and implement ways to improve the operation will not evolve but will stagnate and eventually be unable to meet the clinical and business challenges of the future.

Process improvement means challenging "the way that things have always been done." Not all process improvement programs will succeed in meeting their goals, but all will produce a positive gain for the organization that is willing to take some risk to improve themselves. Through the use of audits, outside reviews, compliance reviews, and just standing back and asking "Why do we do this process this way?" an organization can identify the key areas where improvements in the operation and life of the practice can be made. Process improvement also requires investment – investment in time and thought to evaluate a system and determine a better way to do the job, and investment in education, for it is through education that leadership for improvement is born.

In the realm of clinical practice, areas for review that may result in process improvement include coding documentation, risk assessments, chart audits, and auditing of compliance with regulatory and payer regulations. Within these areas, specific types of audits, reviews, and assessments can include:

1. Reviewing medical records to evaluate completeness of documentation and to identify those providers whose documentation either does not support the procedural code used or who are using a procedural code that is lower than the documentation can support;

2. Comparing the compliance requirements of the various regulatory agencies and third-party payers that use guidelines and policies to ensure the practice meets the expectations of these outside entities; and

3. Reviewing and analyzing the historical data of the organization (e.g., malpractice claims, patient complaints, and external evaluations) to identify trends and areas for additional review and analysis.

All of these reviews can be used as part of larger outcome-based quality assurance programs, which in turn give rise to and support many process improvement initiatives. The vital components of a quality assurance program are structure, process, and outcome, which constitute the framework for quality assurance activities and provide the operational focus for them. Clearly, no one method of measurement has yet evolved as a sole standard of measurement.[3] In most cases, these areas are first addressed through the use of the various audits and assessments. Within larger organizations, these audits can be done internally, assuming qualified personnel exist within the practice; in other cases, these reviews can be contracted out to qualified consultants who can provide the same data at low cost to the practice.

The findings, which reflect on the current structure, process, and outcomes of the services of the organization, are often presented to senior clinical and administrative management for review and corrective action. Without proper and effective communication to all stakeholders, the value of these findings is greatly diminished.

To be most effective, communication of these findings should be provided in written format, but within the context of a face-to-face meeting where effective discussion can take place.

These findings, if utilized properly, become the basis for implementing the various methodologies that may be applied to improve the processes within the organization, including:

1. Flowcharting the process being reviewed to identify possible redundancies or blockages within the process;

2. Reviewing historical data that may exist from previous assessments, such as chart audits, coding reviews, and risk assessments, and comparing those data to current data to identify variations and possible trends that will spotlight concerns and issues; and

3. Completing surveys of patient, referring physician, and employee satisfaction levels to identify issues of concern to these groups of stakeholders.

These methodologies are useful in identifying issues, areas for improvement, and possible systemic changes to the processes in effect. It is often advisable to test the changes through the use of pilot programs before implementing the changes on an organization-wide basis. Through application on a limited scale, an organization is able to test the proposed changes to ensure that there are no unanticipated ramifications emanating from them. After these changes are proven through a pilot program, they can be applied safely throughout the organization.

In order to properly apply and maximize the effect of these reviews within the organization, it is necessary to create teaching models and techniques that effectively impart this knowledge to the staff of the organization. These models vary significantly, based on several factors, including the size of the organization, the existing staff mix, the complexity of the changes that are being envisioned, and the amount of time that can be made available for training and education purposes.

In small organizations, this training can consist of staff meetings, with senior physicians and management providing the training through the use of lectures and roundtable discussions. In larger practices, this training and education may be expanded to include department-specific classes, use of online training programs, and sending staff members to off-site courses and seminars. Without this training and support from senior management and physicians, it is very difficult, if not impossible, to obtain staff buy-in to these new process improvements. It is through this investment in time and resources that an organization will be able to realize improvements in their processes and their clinical outcomes.

■ Capitation Contracting

Capitation contracting is a form of contracting that is fraught with potential exposures. There are basically two types of capitation contracts, each of which has its own set of exposures. With delegated capitation contracts, the provider receives the monthly capitation allowance in advance and uses it to pay for services provided. The advantages of this type of contract are that the practice manages the time delay between the receipt of monies and services provided, and it creates a more timely access to funds. At the same time, however, delegated capitation contracts can create a cash-flow problem for the provider organization, which must be able to cover any member's medical costs within the constraints of the monthly allocation. By contrast, in a nondelegated capitation contract, the managed care plan functions more as a traditional health insurer and pays for services as they are provided. At the end of the agreed-upon contract period, the practice and the plan reconcile the performance and settle the monies.[4] Both methods have benefits and drawbacks, and they both require quality assurance and utilization oversight.

Capitation contracts should be read very carefully with an eye to protection of the rights of patients and the practice. In addition to the financial considerations in the contract review, factors related to quality assurance and patient satisfaction considerations include:

- Services covered under the plan and considerations for how the organization will provide or address services that are not covered with patients;

- Credentialing requirements for providers and peer review considerations;

- Contractual inducements for limiting care, and the organization's processes for ensuring that financial inducements to limit care do not take precedence over the provision of quality care;

- Contract termination duties to the managed care organization and the provider organization's policy and plan for treating and/or transferring patients covered under the plan without risking abandonment or patient dissatisfaction;

- The managed care plan's desired access to records (both medical and business);

- Actual cost to the practice to treat patients in the rated categories vs. the rate being paid per patient;

- Liability and hold-harmless clauses (e.g., the insurer attempting to shift liability for any action or nonaction on its part to the practice); and

- Whether the extent to which the conflict resolution process is delineated by the contract disadvantages the provider in relation to providing care to the patient.[5]

◼ Federal and State Laws and Standards Regarding Industry

Quality processes are governed by a variety of industry regulations and standards. In addition to the surveys provided by the Joint Commission on Accreditation of Healthcare Organizations (JCAHO), the Centers for Medicare and Medicaid Services and other accrediting and state agencies may monitor the health care organization for quality. The medical practice examiner should be knowledgeable about the specific organizations that conduct surveys and audits in the states where the practice has facilities. Whoever interfaces with regulatory agencies should remain apprised of changing regulatory information. This individual often seeks interpretation of regulation as it applies to the specific practices of the medical group, and distributes findings and works with the quality improvement process to facilitate change.

Peer review laws in many states protect quality records from discovery in an effort to ensure free communication about potential issues within the practice. Within that protection, peer review activity, credential files, and event reports are often considered protected information. In addition, many states have legislation and regulations that require reporting specified data elements for state monitoring. Some states are tracking specific disease categories; others may be monitoring treatment processes for specific diagnoses. Each state has its own specific laws regarding protection and reporting with which the medical practice executive involved in risk management activities must be familiar.

◢ Malpractice Risks

Malpractice risks emerge in a variety of ways. Physicians who are incompetent or impaired are a grave danger to the practice for several reasons. Negligent credentialing and negligent hiring are potential allegations. An obvious risk is an untoward event involving patient injury. The reputation of the organization is also at risk because of the perceived tacit approval or acceptance of incompetent or impaired physicians. Although each of these risks is significant, incompetent physicians are not the only malpractice exposure. Poor prescription-writing techniques, including the use of unapproved abbreviations, indiscriminant prescribing of controlled drugs, or illegible handwriting, are significant risks of malpractice as well as patient safety issues.

Physicians who routinely perform unnecessary procedures, either through erroneous clinical judgment or in an effort to maintain productivity levels, are a malpractice risk as well as a fraud and abuse risk. Diagnostic errors and their corresponding consequences, missed diagnoses, and misdiagnoses – all of which can lead to delayed or inappropriate treatment – are major sources of malpractice allegations. Often these types of errors are the result of human factors that contribute to missing a process or not recognizing a vital piece of information. Often, providers receive training in managing procedures and care in accurate and well-managed situations. Simulation and practice are generally inadequate, however, for managing emergencies or for handling the human interaction after unanticipated outcomes. In addition, equipment failure, often unrecognized as such and attributed to human error, as well as other unanticipated hazards, such as a patient falling from an examination table, can create allegations of malpractice. In fact, any number of conditions can contribute to an allegation of malpractice. Nevertheless, three defining factors contribute to whether litigation will be pursued and the outcome of such litigation:

1. The ultimate decision to sue is based on unmet expectations and poor communication between the provider (and staff) and the patient and/or the patient's family.[6]

2. Patients expect honesty and transparent communication.[7]

3. Documentation is a key factor on how well the suit can be defended. As the risk management mantra states, "If it isn't written, it didn't happen."[8]

◼ Medical Service Delivery System

Diminished patient satisfaction results partially from the way health care is delivered. Patients want respect, as do those who deliver care. Waiting times, the method for making appointments, how reliably and efficiently patients flow through the system, and how rushed patients feel during appointments all affect the discrepancy between patient expectations and experience. This discrepancy is what evolves into dissatisfaction such that when something even minor goes wrong during care, the stage is set for anger and disappointment.[9]

Despite temptations to overbook patients to accommodate failures to show, a more realistic scheduling process that allows for variability in visit length based on need is ideal. Recognizing that the ideal will not always be met, a process for communicating with patients about delays in appointments or changes of schedule can address patient needs for timeliness and communication.

The patient flow process, just as any care process, should be diagrammed and evaluated for areas of potential communication failures, information "falling through cracks" in the system, and sources of patient dissatisfaction. The evaluation should consider such issues as time allotment per patient, management of walk-ins and emergencies, processes for appointment making, follow-up appointments, registration, and waiting room environment and time. Resources regarding patient flow are available through the Institute for Healthcare Improvement[10] as well as other sources.

▆ Quality Improvement and the Effective Medical Group

Quality of service provided by group practices is paramount to group practice operations and the future of health care, and, because of increased criticism of health care services, pay for performance is becoming a reality. Quality of service starts with an understanding of what the medical group is really about.

In the past, organizing for delivery of quality was not a central theme for the medical group. Many structural and operational considerations took precedence over quality of care because quality was taken for granted. The lack of standardization, the absence of any formal adherence to best practices, and the lack of formalized quality improvement for programs all contribute to a lack of progress in this area.

Medical group structures are not designed, or in some cases are antithetically designed, to invest in quality initiatives. The ultra-short-term focus of financial performance is a chief culprit. Groups do not invest enough, either financially or in the training needed to carry out large-scale improvement initiatives. Investment dollars come only from the shareholders' pockets, a prospect that has long curtailed the development of modern medical groups.

In his book *Out of the Crisis*,[11] W. Edwards Deming asks a question that should serve as the cornerstone of any group's quality initiative:

> What are you doing about the quality that you hope to provide to your customers four years from now?

The issue of quality in the U.S. health care system is becoming increasingly important as the issue of quality gains more understanding. For most of history, quality has been virtually undefined. As Plato would have said, it is indeed in the eye of the beholder. However, that is changing dramatically and will continue to do so as measures and expectations of quality of health care services continue to evolve.

Team Building

The process of team building is hardly a mystery. Effective team building is an essential responsibility of management and the governance structure of the medical group. Team building and a team-building culture must be developed because it is antithetical to the physician mentality – physicians are trained to work as individuals and to take personal accountability for their actions.

Interactions

Members of a group's governing body must be aware of their own personality and style and how they interact with one another. This is best achieved through personality testing and self-awareness training. The better the team understands its members' individual personalities and leadership styles, and, in general, how they interact with others, the better the team will be at organizational dynamics. For example, dominant personalities become very active when under pressure, which explains why meetings with a number of dominant personalities can often end with argument, conflict, and ultimate indecision. The same skills that may make for a great physician may be useless in the boardroom. Board and general group retreats are excellent ways to improve group dynamics.

Education

Annual retreats can provide educational opportunities, with a choice of topics, such as governance, leadership, business planning, benchmarking, best practices, group dynamics, policy, and legal issues, to focus on each year. In addition, courses, symposia, and other outside sources provide educational opportunities if physicians are given support to attend, meaning time as well as money. The group must encourage and value the development of leaders and demonstrate this by providing resources for the purpose.

In addition, the medical practice executive or other leader can provide an educational presentation at each group meeting, with all levels of staff. Presentations done in Microsoft *PowerPoint*® can then be distributed to the group so any of the members can review the material or see it if they were unable to be at the presentation. An opportunity to discuss the material with group members is also a good idea. Examples of issues for such presentations are the Health Insurance Portability and Accountability Act of 1996 (HIPAA), Medicare and managed care contracts, and Medical Group Management Association data.

Other successful educational activities include:

- A lending library of books and periodicals available to the group members;
- Several copies of a relevant book distributed to the group; and
- Regular e-mails of pertinent articles sent to the group.

Feedback

Processes that are logical and allow participation and input, such as nominal group techniques, surveys, interviews, and planned feedback, can determine whether the practice's team-building activities are welcome and have the desired outcome.

Empowering Teams

One of the greatest deficiencies in group practice administration is physicians' lack of business training and education. This includes the physicians-at-large in the group, as well as those in the governing body. Physician leaders must be groomed, trained, mentored, and educated in the key elements of business success for the medical practice, including working as a team. As with any good orientation program, the assumption is that no one knows anything about governance or how they should behave or function as board members.

The fundamentals of empowering a team are to value team members and their input and to thank the team members regularly, not just when they "leap over tall buildings." Recognition of the team, financially and otherwise, is an important part of team empowerment. Assessment of the team should be part of the performance appraisal process. Celebrate successes as a team in some fun activity. Celebrations can be as simple as a pizza party or they can involve community activities, such as working on a Habitat for Humanity house, volunteering with United Way, participating in an American Heart Association Heart Walk, or helping in a hospital fundraiser.

Chapter 2 **Managing Patient Satisfaction and Customer Service Programs**

◢ Quality Management and Utilization Management

A goal of patient care is to provide the best care and just the right amount of it. Quality management and utilization management processes within the practice have tremendous impact on the cost of services and the outcomes. Triggers for quality management should include any of the exposures in patient care identified during the quality assessment. Each is a potential quality area where patient care is compromised. Furthermore, standard triggers for quality review include sentinel events, repeat admissions within 30 days, and health care–acquired infections, among others. Issues of quality are identified in many ways. Standard event reports and patient complaints are sources of quality information. Furthermore, billing denials and attorney letters of inquiry provide clues to issues of utilization or quality care. Quality improvement should not be a reactive function in postproblem identification, but rather a proactive part of the quality management process to identify problems before they become events.

For quality to be an integral part of the care process, staff must be trained to recognize and report both actual events and situations where systems or processes result in compromised patient safety or care. The organization must have an infrastructure that supports ongoing process improvement through dedicated staff who are trained in process improvement techniques including root cause analysis and failure modes and effects analysis, as well as through resources for making and monitoring recommended changes.

Utilization management ties into the quality process through monitoring practice patterns and patient visits and admissions. Outlier practice patterns, variation in service patterns, and changes in admission and discharge patterns are all indicators of potential quality or process concerns.

■ Patient Satisfaction

Patient satisfaction is a time-honored, long-appreciated, but not often a well-understood factor considered in the improvement of care. Although patient-satisfaction surveys query specific issues such as waiting room time, politeness of staff, or even parking convenience, these surveys primarily measure satisfaction with human interaction. From a patient's perspective, care that is given respectfully and communicated well is care that is appreciated and well perceived.[12] Patient satisfaction measurement tools can provide great feedback for areas in which improvement in quality of processes can be applied, and where staff training on communication and interaction with patients and families will improve the overall relationship of the practice to its customers, patients, and families.

Many organizations use standardized surveys, available from vendors, such as Press Ganey, which allow for benchmarking against similar practices. Nonetheless, simple tools and phone surveys often yield even more pertinent and effective information. In addition to the traditional and important amenity queries about parking, staff politeness, timeliness, and facility, effective satisfaction surveys will measure perceptions of care appropriateness, thoroughness, and communication. In addition, queries about perception of safety and patient involvement in decision making are emerging as a result of the increased focus on patient safety and patient-centered care.

The goal of gathering data is to use it to make change. Patient satisfaction data are useless, however, unless they are used. Properly analyzed, such data hold the key to patient retention and reduced likelihood of litigation. Whatever the methods used by the organization to gather information about patient satisfaction, they should be used to spur change and pinpoint areas for improvement on an ongoing basis.

Data trends should be distributed to appropriate departments and individuals for corrective responses or celebrations of success. Such trends indicate where appropriate quality improvement efforts should be initiated. Customer service training, training in patient-centered care, patient flow processes, or other initiatives can all be monitored through response trends in patient satisfaction surveys. In all cases the data should be communicated with leadership and the board in addition to all staff at least quarterly.

For more about patient satisfaction surveys, refer to the book *Body of Knowledge Review: Patient Care Systems*.

Chapter 3 **Benchmarking Practice Performance**[13]

To compare is to improve.
                    – Unknown

Simply put, benchmarking is measurement and comparison for the purpose of improvement. In particular, medical practice benchmarking is a systematic, logical, and common-sense approach to measurement, analysis, comparison, and improvement (see Exhibit 1). Therefore, benchmarking is comparison to a standard. Benchmarking improves understanding of processes and clinical and administrative characteristics at a single point in time (snapshot) or over time (trend).[14]

In addition, benchmarking is the continuous process of measuring and comparing performance internally (over time) and externally (against other organizations and industries). Finally, benchmarking is determining how the "best in class" achieve their performance levels. This consists of analyzing and comparing best practices to uncover what they did, how they did it, and what must be done to adapt it to your practice (process benchmarking).[15]

◢ Who Set the Standard?

The importance of having a standard is to ensure consistency, a common understanding, and continuity over

---

EXHIBIT 1

What Is Benchmarking?

- A systematic, logical, and common-sense approach to measurement, comparison, and improvement.

- Copying the best, closing gaps and differences, and achieving superiority.[16]

- "A positive, proactive process to change operations in a structured fashion to achieve superior performance. The purpose is to gain a competitive advantage."[17]

- Comparing organizational performance to the performance of other organizations.[18]

- Continuous process of comparison with the best[19] or "the toughest competitors or companies renowned as leaders."[20]

- A method for identifying processes to new goals with full support of management.[21]

---

time. To date, a true standard has not been set for medical practice benchmarking. Therefore, this book is an attempt to rectify this void. In addition, the Medical Group Management Association (MGMA) has a long history of surveying and providing medical practices with valuable benchmarking information. Therefore, survey reports from MGMA are excellent standard-setting (benchmarking) tools because they amass several decades of medical practice data and provide the foundation for building true standards.

Reasons for Benchmarking

There are many reasons for benchmarking.[22] First, benchmarks can be used to objectively evaluate performance to aid in understanding a practice's strengths and weaknesses. Second, benchmarks can be used to observe where a practice has been and predict where it is going. Third, benchmarks can be used to analyze what others have done (best in class) and learn from their experiences (lessons learned). Fourth, benchmarks can be used to determine how the best in class achieve their performance levels and what methods they used to implement their processes. Fifth, benchmarks can be used to convince physicians and staff of the need for change. And sixth, benchmarking can help identify areas for improving practice operations and the bottom line.

When instituting process improvement, benchmarking can uncover areas with the most potential for improvement. In most instances, benchmarking can be considered a method for comparing similar or best practices. In addition, benchmarking is an excellent tool for uncovering different processes and clinical and administrative activities and factors. Also, benchmarking provides valuable, and in most cases, quantitative support to aid in communication, decision-making, and developing buy-in. And in summary, benchmarking can be used to evaluate, observe, analyze, determine best in class, and convince others of a need for change.[23]

The benefits and reasons for benchmarking are to:[24]

- Increase understanding of practice operations;
- Learn about industry leaders, competitors, and best practices;
- Incorporate best practices;
- Gain or maintain a competitive advantage and industry superiority;
- Adopt best practices from any industry into organizational processes (learn and compare against others);
- Break down reluctance to change;
- Uncover new concepts, ideas, and technologies;
- Objectively evaluate performance strengths and weaknesses;
- Observe where you have been and predict where you are going;
- Analyze what others do, to learn from their experiences;
- Determine how the best in class achieve their performance levels so you can implement their processes; and
- Convince internal audiences of the need for change.

■ The "Value" of Benchmarking

Proper benchmarking consists of more than simple comparison of two numbers. The true value of benchmarking lies in the numbers combined with an understanding of the current state of the practice, calculation of the difference between the current state and a new value or benchmark, knowing the context and background of the practice values when interpreting the results, deciding on a course of action and goal, and determining when the goal is achieved. For example, a comparison of average number of procedures per patient visit per physician to a known benchmark will only permit a mathematical analysis. However, what if one physician in the practice has been focusing on patients with simple medical issues that don't generate multiple procedures? The numbers alone would indicate this physician is underperforming and is below the others in procedural productivity; whereas knowing the background, context, or other measures permit for a more detailed analysis. Perhaps this physician's focus is on acute care services and his or her average number of patient encounters per day is almost twice that of other physicians in the practice?

■ Sources of Benchmarks

Benchmarks are available from many sources. The most common benchmarking measures are averages (means) and medians of health care performance measures derived from surveys, reports, or data files. For example, the *MGMA Physician Compensation and Production Survey* and *Cost Survey for Single-Specialty and Multispecialty Practices* are excellent sources for benchmarks. Another source is measures and processes from better-performing practices, which are modeled on organizations that have achieved a particular goal or attained a certain level of success or performance. For instance, the MGMA *Performance and Practices of Successful Medical Groups* is an ideal source for better-performing practice benchmarks. In addition, benchmarks from "best in industry" practices are excellent sources for measures and processes. These benchmarks are taken from organizations inside and outside health care. Of note, benchmarks from outside the health care industry are excellent sources that are often overlooked. For example, the Disney Corporation is a great resource for customer service, and Wal-Mart is ideal for supply-chain management and cost containment.

How to Benchmark

There are several methods of benchmarking.[25] A simple 10-step process might consist of the following:

1. Determine what is critical to your organization's success;
2. Identify metrics that measure the critical factors;
3. Identify a source for internal and external benchmarking data.
4. Measure your practice's performance;
5. Compare your practice's performance to the benchmark;
6. Determine if action is necessary based on the comparison;
7. If action is needed, identify the best practice and process used to implement it;
8. Adapt the process used by others in the context of your practice;
9. Implement new process, reassess objectives, evaluate benchmarking standards, and recalibrate measures; and
10. Do it again – benchmarking is an ongoing process, and tracking over time allows for continuous improvement.

Standardizing Data for Comparison

Because the primary purpose of benchmarking is comparison, it is necessary to standardize data so organizations of different sizes can be compared.[26] A common method for standardizing data is to convert measures to percentages, per unit of input or per unit of output. For example, per unit of input can be presented as per full-time-equivalent (FTE) physician, per FTE provider, or per square foot; whereas, per unit of output can be presented on a per patient, per resource-based relative value scale unit, or per procedure level.

What's Our Baseline?

Like any activity involving comparison, benchmarking requires an understanding of "where you are" – this is known as your baseline. The baseline represents where you are today or where you've been and provides a point of origin or starting point. In addition, a baseline is an initial state that forms a logical basis for comparison.[27] For example, to determine whether physicians have increased the average number of procedures per patient visit, it is necessary to have two measurements: the old value, or baseline, and the new value. To calculate the delta (or difference) between the two values, a simple formula can be used: new value minus old value. Without the baseline, it would not be possible to perform this or many other calculations such as percent change.

How Are We Doing?

This question can be answered by asking the question: "What is the difference between the baseline and your current state (or where we are today)?" The baseline can be an internal benchmark (historical measure) from inside the practice, a benchmark across like practices from an MGMA survey report, or a benchmark from outside the industry such as Disney or Wal-Mart. Additional insights can also be assessed by calculating the difference between your current state and an established benchmark or industry average or median. To determine the difference, there are several methods and statistical tools. For instance, the mathematical difference or delta consists of subtracting the baseline value from the current value, whereas percent change is a method for assessing changes over time or the proportion of one value in comparison to another. In addition to these methods, there are more statistically intense methods for determining difference that can be generalized across a group (see Exhibit 2).

EXHIBIT 2

What Is the Difference?

Mathematical difference (delta)

- New value minus old value;
- Current state minus initial state; and
- Benchmark or industry value minus current state.

Percent change

Inferential statistical methods

Independent T-test

- Difference between two independent averages;

Mann-Whitney U-test

- Difference between two independent medians;

Paired T-test

- Difference between two averages; and
- Comparison of (1) case and matched control or (2) repeated measures.

Wilcoxon Matched Pairs Test

- Difference between two medians;

One-Way ANOVA

- Difference between three or more averages;

Kruskal-Wallis H-test

- Difference between three or more medians.

More complex inferential methods are available to determine the statistical significance of the difference between two or more averages or medians: Independent T-test, Mann-Whitney U-test, Paired T-test, Wilcoxon Matched Pairs Test, One-Way ANOVA (analysis of variance) and Kruskal-Wallis H-test. However, these methods

EXHIBIT 3

Sources of Statistics Information

- Bluman, A.G., *Elementary Statistics: A Step by Step Approach*, 4th ed. Boston: McGraw-Hill, 2001.

- Daniel, W.W., *Biostatistics: A Foundation for Analysis in the Health Sciences*, 7th ed. New York: John Wiley & Sons, 1999.

- Kelley, L.D., *Measurement Made Accessible: A Research Approach Using Qualitative, Quantitative, and Quality Improvement Methods.* Thousand Oaks, CA: SAGE Publications, 1999.

- Rosner, B., *Fundamentals of Biostatistics*, 3rd ed. Boston: PWS-Kent Publishing Company, 1990.

- Rothstein, J.M., and J.L. Echternach, *Primer on Measurement: An Introductory Guide to Measurement Issues.* Alexandria, VA: American Physical Therapy Association, 1993.

- Tabachnick, B.G., and L.S. Fidell, *Using Multivariate Statistics*, 4th ed. Boston: Allyn and Bacon, 2001.

require greater understanding of the use, limitations, requirements, analysis and interpretation of each technique, and are outside the scope of this book. For information on these methods, see Exhibit 3 for a short list of resources.

Interpretation of the difference is dependent on the method used. When using the delta, the difference will be a raw number, because the method consists of simple subtraction. Determining whether the difference is good or bad depends on the context, background, and what the values represent. For example, if medical revenue after operating cost per FTE family practice physician is $145,000 and the MGMA benchmark indicates a median of $214,377, then the delta is $69,377 ($214,377 minus $145,000). A delta of $69,377 may suggest poor practice performance, reduced physician productivity, a capital investment or other practice deficiencies, or large expenses. On the

EXHIBIT 4

Difference Between Delta and Percent Change

Is the Result Positive or Negative?	Delta	Percent Change
Positive value	New value (or bench-mark) is greater than the old value.	New value has *increased*.
	For example, $214,377 minus $145,000 equals a delta of $69,377.	For example, $145,000 divided by $214,377 equals 0.67 and when multiplied by 100 equals 67 percent.
Negative value	New value is less.	New value has *decreased*.

other hand, the percent change method indicates this practice is only generating 67 percent of the median for similar types of practices (see Exhibit 4). Therefore, the result is different between delta and percent change, and the interpretation may also be different.

Getting from Here to There

When the difference between baseline and current state or current state and benchmark is known, the next step is to determine, first, whether there is a desire to change and, second, what factors (practice measures) can be influenced in the preferred direction. Therefore, it is imperative that a desire to change be established throughout the organization. In addition, it should be grown and nurtured by involving physicians and staff in the entire process.

EXHIBIT 5

Resources for Best Practices and Lessons Learned

■ MGMA's EBSCO (Elton B. Stephens Company) database*	■ The McKinsey Quarterly (www.mckinseyquarterly.com)
■ MGMA e-mail forums*	■ Harvard Business Review (www.hbr.org)
■ MGMA assemblies and societies*	■ Six Sigma (www.isixsigma.com)
* Require MGMA membership.	

■ Best Practices and Lessons Learned

Knowing the best method for completing a task and the mistakes to avoid would result in quicker and less costly improvements. Lessons learned are suggested techniques or efficiencies for overcoming errors or avoiding mistakes. They can be tips, tricks, or cautions from those who have already tried and succeeded (or failed). And best practices are specific characteristics, measures, or processes considered to be best in class by subjective (personal opinion) or objective criteria (for example, a measure at or above the 90th percentile). Exhibit 5 presents a short list of resources for finding best practices and lessons learned.

■ Methods and Checklists

Failing to plan, it has been said, is planning to fail. Therefore, an integral component of the benchmarking process is the proper use of systematic methods, checklists, scales, and comparable measures. Systematic methods consist of formulas and ratios. Checklists are a

---

EXHIBIT 6

Example Checklist[28]

The following checklist items can be used to increase the likelihood that a claim will be processed and paid when first submitted:

☐ Patient information is complete.

☐ Patient's name and address matches the insurer's records.

☐ Patient's group number and/or subscriber number is correct.

☐ Physician's Social Security number, provider number, or tax identification number is completed and correct.

☐ Claim is signed by the physician.

☐ All necessary dates are completed.

☐ Dates for care given are chronological and correct. For example, is the discharge date listed as occurring before the admission date?

☐ Dates for care given are in agreement with the claims information from other providers such as the hospital, etc.

☐ Diagnosis is complete.

☐ Diagnosis is correct for the services or procedures provided.

☐ Diagnostic codes are correct for the services or procedures provided.

☐ CPT® and ICD-9 codes are accurate.

☐ Diagnosis is coded using ICD-9-CM to the highest level of specificity.

☐ Fee column is itemized and totaled.

☐ All necessary information about prescription drugs or durable medical equipment prescribed by the physician is included.

☐ The claim is legible.

---

planning tool to ensure that all variables and methods are used and considered – checklists ensure attention to detail and minimize the chance of missing steps in a process (see Exhibit 6). Scales provide the measuring stick – meaning they indicate whether your measures are high or low, good or bad, or where they are in comparison to others. And comparable measures are key to the heart and soul of benchmarking and provide a means for determining how your practice compares to others.

■ Small and Solo Practice Benchmarking

Small and solo practices share many similarities with their larger counterparts; however, the benefits and risks associated with the differences can have significant impact on a small practice's longevity and financial success.

■ Similarities with Larger Practices

All medical practices must operate in the same health care environment and deal with the same health care legislation, malpractice insurance, payers, collection challenges, patient needs and expectations, delivery and standards of care, and processes – just to name a few. Also, the benchmarking methods used by large organizations are identical to those used by small and solo practices (see Exhibit 7). And the use of standardized metrics permits comparison regardless of organizational size. Common examples available in most benchmarking data sets consist of measures per FTE physician/provider, per square foot, per patient, per procedure, and per relative value unit (RVU).[29]

■ What's the Difference?

Small and solo practices are different from larger groups in several ways, some of which are beneficial, while others are not. For instance, smaller organizations are generally more flexible, can adapt and change quickly, and, in general, tend to be more efficient. However, small and solo practices are more sensitive to the risks associated with costly mistakes, lack of alternative revenue-generating methods, and the absence of (or antiquated condition of) robust information systems. For example, with only one or two physicians in a practice, what impact would a poor decision or loss of a physician (due to sickness or some other unforeseen event) have on the practice? Can

EXHIBIT 7

Similarities Regardless of Practice Size or Type[30]

- Legislation can change payment (for example, Medicare/Medicaid reimbursement rates are determined through legislation).

- Costs are increasing greater than inflation (for example, medical supplies and equipment costs are increasing at a greater percentage than reimbursement rates).

- Expenses change.

- Increases in physician compensation are from production (for example, much of physician compensation is based on physician production, or the number of patients seen and the procedures performed).

- Health savings accounts will change patient behavior (for example, patients will treat medical care more like a product or service they pay for using funds in their account).

- Hospitals are purchasing physician practices (again).

- Advances in medical care are changing care delivery.

- Physicians are publicly rated for quality and outcomes.

- Physicians are publicly rated for patient satisfaction.

a small practice afford to retain adequate earnings for contingencies? Does the existing information system complement and add to the efficiency of the practice? And does it interface (communicate) with the information systems used by payers, hospitals, and other medical practices such as referring practices and physicians?

Ultimately, the goals of smaller practices mirror those of larger groups – to have more satisfied patients, more fulfilling work environments for physicians and staff, and better economic outcomes.[31] However, the additional sensitivities of small and solo practices must be considered to ensure that surprise events don't adversely impact the practice.

■ Industry Quality Benchmarks

Medical group practice quality initiatives should be led and pas-
sionately promoted by the governance structures of the group. A
pay-for-performance program, accreditation, malpractice concerns,
and consumer demand all work to create an increasing expectation
of continually improving patient care that can be demonstrated
by objective data and systematic measurement. The National
Committee for Quality Assurance (NCQA) has led this effort for
more than two decades. Activities include many quality initiatives
focused on practice profiles, practice guidelines based on evidence-
based data, education of practitioners, and health plans for patients.
The Healthcare Effectiveness Data and Information Set (HEDIS)
report evaluates health plans through measurement of their specific performance in a number of quality areas, such as prevention,
screening of patients, and other clinical measures.

Practices may seek accreditation by providing data about their
activities including clinical measures required by NCQA that are
submitted during the accreditation process.[32]

Satisfaction Surveys

Satisfaction surveys are essential for evaluating an organization and
are a cornerstone of quality improvement programs. For satisfaction surveys to be successful, a number of factors are important.
Surveying is a widely studied area. A great deal of information is
available to help guide the surveying strategy of the group.

- *The testing should be simple and reproducible.* This is an activity that may be worth outsourcing to a testing company
  that can provide survey tools and analysis.

- *Concerns that are identified in the survey should be addressed.*
  Surveys should not ask about things that the practice is not
  prepared to address because that will only create additional
  dissatisfaction. This may also be true for issues that the
  practice may not have control over, such as patients' health
  plans. Patient satisfaction does correlate to health plans, but
  the practice has little opportunity to address those issues.

- *The questions should be simple, direct, and short.* This is especially true of general surveys. Focus groups or more in-depth surveys may be appropriate when addressing specific issues (e.g., the need for evening and weekend hours).

- *The validity of the questions should be examined through statistical analysis.* In other words, question outcomes should actually correlate with satisfaction.

- *The practice should design specific interventions for problem areas* and use these plans as opportunities to educate the staff and physicians.

- *Surveys should be repeated on a regular schedule and the results tracked over time.* This will help to evaluate intervention success. Satisfaction is a matter for the entire group, not just the administration, governing board, or the physicians, so this information should be shared with everyone in the organization.

Benchmark Tracking

Although performance measurements are covered very well in other volumes in the *Medical Practice Management Body of Knowledge* series, benchmarking, preparation of dashboards, and report cards are some of the best ways for the governing body of the group to monitor organizational goals. Benchmarks produce a quick, easy-to-understand, and high-impact way to communicate essential information.

It is important to develop a series of benchmarks that can be tracked over time to monitor the progress and status of the group performance. This will include quality indicators, such as results of quality initiatives, comparisons with peer databases, and financial indicators such as:

- Gross revenue/per RVU;
- Collections/per RVU;
- Profit/net income/per RVU;

EXHIBIT 8.
Sample Quarterly Report – Three-Year Comparison

	1st Qtr 2006 Conversion Factor: 36.3167 Total RVUs = 303,264		1st Qtr 2007 Conversion Factor: 38.2581 Total RVUs = 324,016		1st Qtr 2008 Conversion Factor: 36.1992 Total RVUs = 316,326	
	Totals	$ Per RVU	Totals	$ Per RVU	Totals	$ Per RVU
Gross Revenue	$12,821,311	$42	$14,918,834	$46	$14,648,065	$46
Collections	12,814,986	42	14,773,024	46	14,405,557	46
Profit/ Net Income	1,765,542	6	2,774,379	9	1,804,222	6
Operating Cost	6,793,882	22	7,602,643	23	8,391,248	27
Employee Salary	2,740,441	9	3,125,846	10	14,918,834	47

Physician Productivity Measures per Quarter

Total RVUs	303,264		324,016		316,326	
	No. of MDs	RVUs per MD	No of MDs	RVUs per MD	No. of MDs	RVUs per MD
	50	6,065	55	5,856	58	5,471

- RVU per physician;
- Operating cost/per RVU; and
- Employee salary/per RVU.

RVUs make excellent measurement tools because they have become a standard part of group practice management and reimbursement systems. They have universal applicability and recognition.[33]

Exhibit 8 is an example of a simple benchmarking report card that can be used by a governing body to monitor organizational performance.

Benchmarks need to be understandable. They must communicate their meaning clearly, be reproducible over time, and be current for quickly reacting to changing situations. Benchmarks also need to measure key competencies or key success indicators for the practice.

In summary, benchmarking allows the governing body to:

- Compare the practice to those of successful peers;[34]
- Communicate in times of rapid change when internal sign-posts are less clear;
- Analyze activity (by using internal and external benchmarks);
- Evaluate specific procedures and processes (e.g., collection, profitability);
- Take action on a specific need or problem; and
- Evaluate change.

Benchmark Characteristics

The key characteristics of benchmarks are that they should be:

- Relevant to the business and measure key indicators that drive profitability, quality, or other critical success factors;
- Timely – old news is no news;
- Able to differentiate between accountable items (e.g., whether each benchmark provides new information);
- Adaptable and adoptable, so physicians and staff can learn from peers; and
- Consistent, using the same metrics each time (e.g., not using RVUs during one period of time, only to change to a dollars-per-unit of service on the next).

Benchmarking Problems

It may be difficult to evaluate the effects of individual variations in processes, variables, and other parameters. It is therefore important that the practice should not expect too much from the benchmarking process; it is not a substitute for good management, it is only a tool.

Surprisingly little profit variation may be explained by the usual causes. This can lead to classic strategic errors in correcting a perceived problem. Therefore, a number of indicators should be considered, and over time those that correlate best with the business will become apparent.

Every governing body faces the challenge of effectively monitoring data about the well-being of the practice without trying to glean this information from raw data or detailed reports. Dashboards and benchmarking report cards are useful for this purpose and can be prepared by the finance department or administration. A detailed review of data should be reserved for areas of concern. By benchmarking key financial and other important practice parameters, the board can effectively monitor the critical activities of practice performance and fulfill this important obligation to the members of the group.

Dashboards

A practice dashboard is a technique that uses simple visual indications of how a particular activity is progressing in absolute terms or in terms relative to a goal. As can be seen in Exhibit 9, this simple representation of positive and negative trends can quickly communicate a great deal of information effectively. This feature is especially useful when meeting time is limited because information presented in this manner reduces the need to interpret detailed reports.

Most medical groups prepare profit-and-loss (P&L) statements on a regular basis. Such financial records and documents are essential and helpful for the medical practice executive, but many do little to guide strategic issues or to plan for the future. Two essential financial planning instruments are the budget and the pro forma financial statement.

The budget provides a financial look into the future based on proposed activities of the group. The budget steps that the medical plan executive follows in preparing the budget for the group are as follows:

Step 1: Perform an environmental assessment and strategic plan review.
Step 2: Establish the budget guidelines.

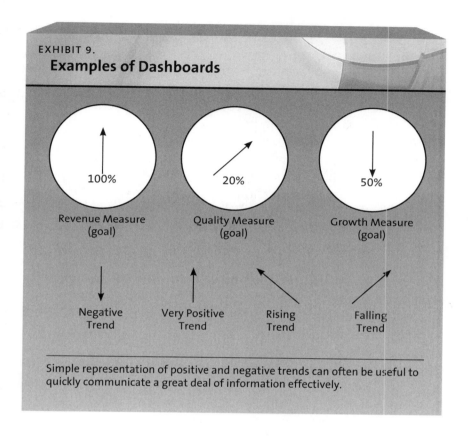

EXHIBIT 9.

Examples of Dashboards

100%

Revenue Measure
(goal)

20%

Quality Measure
(goal)

50%

Growth Measure
(goal)

Negative
Trend

Very Positive
Trend

Rising
Trend

Falling
Trend

Simple representation of positive and negative trends can often be useful to quickly communicate a great deal of information effectively.

Step 3: Provide detailed forecasts, and historical and comparative information.

Step 4: Review forecast against the guidelines.

Step 5: Revise as necessary.

Step 6: Submit to board for presentation and approval.

The pro forma financial statement is essentially an estimate of the profit and loss from a particular service or proposed activity. It would involve all of the steps that are necessary for preparing a P&L statement, but in most cases, much of the information is estimated based on what is expected.

Modeling

Although budgets and pro formas essentially are financial models of the medical group as a whole (budget) or of a particular service (pro forma), more specific modeling data can be developed to guide practice planning and development. The medical practice executive should understand the concepts of variable costs, fixed costs, and revenue data. For example, if one were to consider opening a satellite office in a new city, many strategic reasons may be important and would contribute to making the decision to open this office, but certainly financial considerations and modeling would be important. If patients and revenue growth are the goals of opening the new office, then a model that allows the enterprise to calculate the number of patients required to generate particular revenue would be important.

Such data can be modeled based on reasonable assumptions, which can be gained from the typical practice management system. For example:

$$\frac{\text{Total Patient Revenue}}{\text{Number of Patients or RVUs}} = \text{Average Patient Revenue}$$

$$\frac{\text{Total Cost}}{\text{Number of Patients or Revenue}} = \text{Average Patient Cost}$$

Assumptions about variables such as age, diagnosis, and time can all be included to help create a forecasting model of a new location or service. Typically, expenses are much easier to forecast than revenue for any practice activity because expenses are more easily identifiable. Other valuable data include the frequency of the service on a national or regional basis and the frequency of the diagnosis on a national or regional basis. Much of these data are available from MGMA.

As electronic patient records and better practice management systems are developed, modeling will become easier, faster, more accurate, and therefore, more useful.

Chapter 4 **Creating Pay-for-Performance Programs to Enhance Health Care Quality**

Pay-for-Performance (P4P) and Physician Compensation[35]

While fee-for-service continues to be the most widely used mechanism to reimburse physicians for professional services, a contingent reimbursement strategy termed "pay-for-performance," also known as "P4P," is emerging as a popular methodology for payers who are seeking a way to foster high-quality, low-cost health care services. P4P programs differentially reimburse physicians based on their achievement of specific clinical and practice efficiency measures. These programs seek to focus physician attention and performance on effective care management and clinical outcomes through the use of discrete measures and incentives. A number of medical practices have extended this reimbursement strategy (payments from health plan to medical practice) to physician compensation plans or incentive plans (payments from medical practice to physician), effectively aligning the reimbursement mechanism that generates revenue to the practice with the payment mechanism that pays physicians for their services.

◾ Background

Historically, medical practices have generally thrown up their hands when the issue of differentiating performance or quality has been raised. Many believed that it was simply too difficult to control for the many idiosyncratic factors that impact quality of patient care – specifically, the patient-specific variables of genetics, age, risk factors, co-morbidities, socioeconomic status, compliance with treatment plans, and other similar factors. Medical practices that sought to differentially reward physicians based on quality thus tended to focus on "proxies" of quality that involved more easily measured issues of medical record documentation (e.g., timeliness and completeness), patient perceptions of service delivery (e.g., derived from patient satisfaction surveys or patient complaint tracking), and patient access (e.g., access to third available appointment and wait time upon presentation for a scheduled appointment).

Today, however, electronic health records (EHRs) and other sophisticated information technologies have facilitated capture, reporting, and analysis of clinical data by medical practices and payers. Many practices have now negotiated terms in their health plan contracts that permit differential reimbursement based on clinical or quality measures. In the past, the measures that were selected for contingent reimbursement tended to focus on those that were readily available to the health plan – data submitted on a billing claim form. Increasingly, however, health plans are requiring additional data to be submitted by medical groups that involve data mining of medical records, self-reports of technological readiness, patient access data, and other similar indices.

◾ The P4P Debate

There are strong proponents and strong detractors of P4P as a reimbursement strategy. Proponents argue that contingent reimbursement will help to more quickly transition the health care industry to a focus on prevention and wellness (which is expected to reduce the cost of care), encourage medical practices to institute EHRs, and permit consumers (employers, health plans, and patients) to differentiate performance of medical practices (and physicians) based on clinical and practice efficiency measures. P4P reimbursement mechanisms are relatively new, and proponents include employers concerned about rising health care costs; health plans seeking to differentiate high-quality, low-cost physicians; and patients who are seeking a high return on investment as they pay rising out-of-pocket expenses for health care services. Proponents tend to view P4P as an alignment strategy (long overdue), aligning the interests of employers, health plans, medical practices, and patients on high-quality, low-cost care.

Those opposing P4P programs tend to not oppose the underlying concepts of P4P arrangements; rather, they question whether the measures that are selected for contingent reimbursement truly define "quality." These individuals are asking questions related to the long-term impact of linking payment to the measures that heretofore have been selected. For example, what is the impact on physicians and medical groups who treat very ill patients? What is the impact on physicians and medical groups that have a large, noncompliant patient base? What is the impact on small practices that do not have the administrative infrastructure to compete for these additional funds? What is the impact on the overall revenue stream for a medical practice as more and more of the dollars are paid in this type of contingent fashion? In general, opponents of P4P are highly skeptical and are concerned that P4P may lead to further declines in reimbursement for professional services, may encourage undue competition, and/or may not result in the high-quality, low-cost outcomes that are anticipated from these programs.

In the future, if P4P comes to represent a large portion of the reimbursement dollar, concerns regarding differential access for specific types of patients and the financial and other impacts on medical practices will need to be addressed. The impact this will have on physician perceptions of clinical autonomy, revenue performance, measures of physician work and effort, and the alignment within internal compensation strategies remains to be seen.

◾ Aligning Compensation with Reimbursement

It is important for a compensation plan to be aligned with the reimbursement mechanism of the medical practice to not only ensure fiscal responsibility but also to optimize revenue performance. For example, if a medical practice has 75 percent of its revenue paid via capitation contracts, a physician compensation plan that rewards physicians based on professional services gross charges or patient visits alone is likely nonsensical. Similarly, if a medical practice generates 75 percent of its revenue via fee-for-service contracts, a compensation plan that only addresses panel size may be misaligned with revenue-generating opportunity. With P4P reimbursement, a similar situation holds. That is, if a significant percentage of the revenue of a medical practice is derived through P4P strategies that predicate reimbursement on specific clinical, patient safety, or practice efficiency measures, a compensation plan based solely on professional services net collections or work relative value units (WRVUs) is likely not aligned with the financial reality that revenue is contingent on measures which extend beyond clinical production.

There does not necessarily need to be a one-to-one relationship between the reimbursement mechanism and the physician compensation mechanism. Some practices, for example, still pay physicians on straight salary arrangements while receiving their revenue via discounted fee-for-service strategies. For purposes of this chapter, the importance of P4P in physician compensation relates to one of alignment. As reimbursement levels from these arrangements increase to represent a significant portion of a practice's revenue, practices will likely attempt to align their internal physician compensation plans in order to ensure heightened focus on these performance criteria to optimize revenue to the medical practice.

◾ P4P Methods and Measures

A number of different compensation strategies are used to recognize and reward physicians for P4P measures. Similarly, a number of different contracting strategies are used to generate P4P dollars. The following sections discuss the P4P methods and measures currently adopted by medical practices.

P4P strategies used in the context of physician compensation take one of three forms: (1) direct; (2) indirect; or (3) integrative treatment of these funds for physician compensation purposes.

1. Direct Treatment

In a direct treatment of P4P dollars, a medical practice adopts a direct "pass-through" approach of these dollars to the physicians who "earned" them, consistent with the P4P contracted measures. In this direct treatment, this payment is above and beyond what the physician receives due to the physician compensation plan that the practice has adopted. In some cases, the practice may retain an administrative fee related to managing the infrastructure to monitor and document performance and/or to contract, manage, and disburse the funds. Otherwise, all P4P dollars are paid directly to the earning physicians.

The advantage of this direct approach to P4P dollars is that physicians who are directly responsible for earning this contingent payment individually benefit from their work – and they also recognize the magnitude of that benefit.

The disadvantages of a direct approach to administering P4P are twofold: (1) the P4P component of compensation may be wholly inconsistent with the internal physician compensation plan, leading to conflicts regarding priorities and focus; and (2) as the amount of revenue grows from P4P in comparison to "traditional" fee-for-service reimbursement, this direct treatment may be inconsistent with the goals of compensating physicians in the practice. In essence, this represents an individualistic, performance-based compensation plan, with the same advantages and disadvantages of these plans, including a lack of team orientation and focus on cost-of-practice issues.

2. Indirect Treatment

In an indirect treatment of P4P dollars, a medical practice generally elects one of three options: (1) to treat P4P dollars as simply another revenue source in the funds flow model that is available for physician compensation purposes, with the overall compensation plan generally silent as to the P4P measures; (2) to create a separate incentive pool for these dollars that may be "earned" by the physicians (including those physicians who did not generate the P4P dollars); or (3) to use the P4P dollars for discretionary purposes.

In the first indirect treatment method, the current internal physician compensation plan is not impacted in a material way; however, the method used to credit physicians for their productivity is extended to these funds as well. So, for example, if a practice credits physicians for net collections from professional services by using a percentage of net collections to total net collections basis, then this same percentage is applied to the P4P dollars received by the practice, with each physician receiving his or her portion consistent with the revenue treatment method identified for professional services.

In the second indirect treatment method involving a separate incentive pool for P4P funds, the money is awarded to physicians based on criteria established by the practice that may or may not have a direct linkage to the measures used to generate the P4P dollars.

When an indirect treatment of these funds is employed, any number of methods may be used to distribute this revenue to physicians, including:

- Per physician (equal share);
- Per physician full-time-equivalent (FTE) (equal share adjusted for FTE);
- Based on individual physician professional services net collections as a percentage of total net collections;
- Based on individual WRVUs as a percentage of total WRVUs; or
- Others.

In the third indirect treatment method, in some cases, the medical practice may elect a discretionary use of these funds consistent with practice needs. For example, it applies these dollars to practice operating expense, thereby reducing overall expenditures specifically allocated to physicians; or it uses the funds to support new program development, to support physician leadership or administrative stipends, or for other purposes in the practice.

The advantage of the indirect treatment of P4P includes the recognition that a group or team orientation (rather than simply individual physician effort) is needed to ensure high-quality, low-cost care for patients (which is what the P4P dollars typically represent). Thus, all of the physicians in the practice have an opportunity to "earn" P4P dollars through additional revenue credit and/or through a new incentive pool option, or the practice as a whole benefits from the additional revenue that has been generated.

The disadvantage of the indirect treatment is the general lack of focus and accountability for performance relative to the P4P measures and its promised revenue potential. Because physicians do not perceive a direct reward for generating the funds, there may be less focus on the measures and outcomes. Of course, this disadvantage can be overcome if the P4P dollars are sufficiently great to warrant collective attention to the performance measures and/or if the practice builds in performance expectations related to program participation.

3. Integrative Treatment

The third strategy involves an "integrative" approach to P4P allocation. In these practices, a larger program of clinical engagement or integration is adopted, with that program funded via the P4P dollars. In this strategy, an overall program to recognize physicians for their high-quality, low-cost outcomes is developed and typically involves multiple measures of performance (often beyond those identified in the contracts with the health plans for these dollars), and typically also applies to all patients (beyond those for which the P4P dollars are derived).

The strategy adopted by a medical practice to compensate physicians involving P4P dollars and measures typically depends on the goals of the compensation plan for a particular medical practice, as well as on the amount of revenue available from P4P-contracted dollars that is used to fund physician compensation.

Because of the perspective it can provide, benchmarking (refer to Chapter 3) is an essential element of the process needed to develop any effective physician compensation plan.

◾ Clinical Pathways

Clinical pathways are described as multidisciplinary plans of treatment that are developed to enable the implementation of clinical guidelines and protocols. While best known as clinical pathways, several other terms are used to describe this concept, including care maps, integrated care pathways, and collaborative care pathways. Clinical pathways are utilized to support clinical, resource, and financial management of a patient with a specific condition over a specified time period. The four major components to the clinical pathway include (1) a time line, (2) the type of care, (3) the outcome criteria, and (4) the variance record for identifying deviations from the norms and/or expectations.[36]

The goal of developing and implementing clinical pathways and clinical protocols is to attain a high level of quality of medical care by identifying, implementing, and adhering to specific medical standards by all physicians in a given specialty when treating a specific set of symptoms or identified illness or injury. Through the application of clinical pathways in the utilization of clinical protocols, a group practice will have the tools to generate clinical data that will enable the organization to prove to outside entities the level of clinical quality being provided by the practice.

Clinical pathways and protocols can be derived from multiple sources, including third-party payers, medical specialty societies, and the National Institutes of Health. Even though applying these protocols constitutes good clinical care on its own, the utilization of audits and external assessments to measure compliance with the protocols can be effectively used to confirm the quality of care being provided and therefore justify the negotiation of better contracts with third-party payers and improved relationships with local employers where direct contracting for medical services may be possible.

The effective development and implementation of clinical pathways within an organization requires a multidisciplinary approach, with input from all levels of clinical providers as well as input from nonclinical staff. The initial creation of this type of structure requires the full and unreserved endorsement and support of physicians as well as clinical and executive leadership of the organization. Preliminary meetings and discussions need to be held within the leadership structure to identify the organization-specific goals for the implementation of clinical pathways. In some cases, this may require the inclusion of various community collaborators who have involvement or responsibility for part of the care and treatment plan of the patient. Examples of this outside collaboration may include visiting-nurse services, rehabilitation facilities, and social services support agencies. In addition to being part of the leadership, administrative support goes further in the form of being advocates, facilitators, and champions to show that the organization is in favor of and supportive of the implementation of clinical pathways through both words and the identification and application of necessary financial and operational resources.

In addition, the development and implementation of clinical pathways may have significant effects that go beyond the simple goal of quality care. The development and application of clinical pathway structures, when properly communicated to staff, patients, and community stakeholders, send a clear and effective message that the practice is committed to maintaining services at no less than industry norms and is effective at both identifying and measuring those norms for improved patient care. Properly designed and implemented clinical pathways will also affect the cost of care through changes in the services that will be rendered based on specific presented symptoms, and may have significant impact on insurance carrier–directed pay-for-performance models. The application of clinical pathways should also increase financial accountability through the elimination of redundancy and variations of clinical methods used by different providers.

In addition to developing and implementing this clinical pathway structure, an organization should create and implement a variety of quality assurance programs to measure the results of the implementation of the clinical pathways and ensure that the desired goals are being reached. The majority of quality assurance programs can be sized to meet the needs of both large and small medical practices. Depending on the size of the organization, some practices complete their quality assurance programs internally whereas other practices utilize outside consultants to complete the necessary reviews, audits, and surveys.

A key tool in evaluating adherence to clinical pathways and their effect on the patient population is through the use of various outcomes measures, including chart reviews, whereby a sample of medical records is reviewed to confirm that the proper care is being provided and properly documented in the medical record. Other measurements that can be used include patient and referring-physician satisfaction surveys. These surveys, when completed properly and analyzed in a timely manner, can provide a wealth of information concerning how well the clinical pathways are being received and whether the pathways are in keeping with the standards in the community and the expectations of the patient. The results of these reviews and surveys should be presented to senior clinical and administrative management to enable them to address the issues raised by the results of the surveys and reviews. The data used to define the issues may be perceived differently when reviewed by clinical and administrative staff. Clinicians will be primarily seeking to improve the care being provided to enable the patient to reach the best possible outcome. This goal is important from the administrative point of review as well, but the medical practice administrator is also concerned that the care and service are being provided in the most cost-effective manner with the most efficient use of available resources. Finally, these data are critical to identifying and determining modifications that need to be made in both the strategic and operational planning processes.

Chapter 5   # Managing Staff, Business, and Equipment Credentialing and Licensure

IN THE PERCEPTION OF THE PUBLIC, the primary reason for accreditation and credentialing is to be able to show that an outside, independent body has determined that an organization (or an individual) has been tested and has met standards that prove its level of quality and/or competency within the health care field.

With regard to organizations and facilities, the primary accrediting bodies are the Joint Commission on Accreditation of Healthcare Organizations and the Accreditation Association for Ambulatory Health Care. When pursuing accreditation, a practice or health care facility should undergo a rigorous multiday evaluation that addresses all aspects of the operation of the organization and the medical treatment that is being provided.

Within this accreditation process, an organization can expect that evaluations of the following areas will take place:

- Governing by-laws;
- Safety and health procedures;

- Facility design and safety;
- Chart documentation;
- Human resources;
- Quality assurance reviews; and
- Physician and staff credentialing.

In addition, the development, implementation, and adherence to documented policies and procedures that delineate and govern the day-to-day operations of the practice are critical to the successful completion of the accreditation process. This in-depth evaluation is repeated, normally on a three-year cycle, to ensure that the findings of both the initial and subsequent evaluations are still within the expected values that earned the organization its original accreditation.

Failure to meet the expected standards places a requirement on the organization to implement corrective action to address those issues that did not meet the standards of the accrediting body. Continued failure to be responsive to and correct these deficiencies can result in increasing levels of response from the accrediting body, with the ultimate response being the revocation of the certificate of accreditation.

In addition to these accreditation organizations, other recognized professional organizations provide the means to credential or certify the competency of physicians and administrators. Physicians obtain their board certification through the completion of specialty training and the successful passing of comprehensive examinations that test their knowledge and expertise within their defined areas of specialization. In many cases, this board certification is required to obtain privileges within hospital staffs and participation on various insurance carrier provider panels. This board certification is specialty-controlled, and retaining this certification normally requires that the physician complete specified numbers of continuing-education credits each year as well as take periodic re-examinations intended to ensure that the physician has remained current with the changes in the field of specialty.

This form of comprehensive testing also is available to h care administrators as a means of confirming their expertise and abil- ity in the field of health care management. The two organizations that are recognized for providing this testing and certification are the American College of Medical Practice Executives (ACMPE) and the American College of Healthcare Executives (ACHE). Whereas ACMPE's primary thrust is in the area of group practice manage- ment, ACHE is the more prevalent credentialing body in the area of hospital administration. Both organizations require that a mem- ber who has attained certification complete a specified number of continuing-education hours in each three-year period to retain the certification designation.

In addition to the professional credentialing organizations pre- viously discussed, physicians are also credentialed by licensed health care facilities (e.g., hospitals and nursing homes) and by commercial and noncommercial insurance carriers. Each organization has its own policies and procedures for credentialing providers and confirming and updating those credentials. Each entity has its own regulations that must be followed by the credentialed provider. In the event of noncompliance with the policies and guidelines of the credentialing body, the provider may be subject to progressive disciplinary action, which ultimately may result in the provider losing credentialed sta- tus with the entity. Normally, the provider is advised of the area of noncompliance and is offered the opportunity to implement cor- rective action within a defined period of time. Failure to implement corrective action or continued violations of the specific policies and procedures may result in progressively stronger disciplinary actions including suspension and ultimate termination from the staff, if a health care facility, or termination from the provider panel, if an insurance carrier.

To properly and effectively manage the myriad regulations, licenses, and credentialing requirements of its health care providers, it is advantageous for the practice to develop a database that reflects and summarizes all of these areas so that the practice's leadership can, at a glance, identify areas of conflict or areas where informa- tion requires updating. A simple way to create such a database is through the use of electronic spreadsheets, which can be updated as information on the individual members of the practice changes. Through the use of spreadsheets, a practice can chart the status of the credentialing of individual providers within a health plan and can maintain an electronic "tickler file" of when various licenses and certifications are due for renewal.

■ Credentialing Process[37]

Prior to officially joining any practice – and in many cases, prior to the interview – physicians will need to complete several credentialing processes. These steps are critical for many legal reasons.

Laws in all 50 states and the District of Columbia establish physician licensure requirements for persons practicing medicine within the jurisdictions. Some jurisdictions also prohibit, either through explicit statements in their medical practice acts or through case law, the so-called corporate practice of medicine. This doctrine generally forbids physicians from practicing medicine on behalf of, or in concert with, any organization other than a professional services corporation (or similar corporate entity) for the practice of medicine. In some states, similar limitations are also imposed, to a greater or lesser degree, on other licensed health care professionals (e.g., psychologists) delivering services in a corporate setting.

Many states have watered down this strict prohibition to allow nonprofit hospital service corporations, health maintenance organizations, and certain other enterprises to employ physicians. For example, some states also allow employers to hire physicians to provide medical services to their own employees and their dependents at company-sponsored clinics. In other jurisdictions, hospital employment may be authorized on the grounds that the delivery of medical care is consistent with the hospital's mission.

Background

For the most part, such prohibitions on the corporate practice of medicine originated in the early 1900s. Several policy concerns underlie the prohibition, including the desire to (1) avoid layperson control over professional medical judgment, (2) prevent commercial exploitation of medical practice, and (3) prevent any conflict between a physician's duty of loyalty to his or her patient and to his or her employer. In many states, physicians who violate the prohibition on the corporate practice of medicine are subject to disciplinary action, including potential loss of their medical license. Directors and officers of organizations who violate the prohibition may also be subject to civil and potentially criminal penalties.

Legal Requirements

To meet these legal requirements, physicians and their practice managers must take many credentialing steps, some of which are required before any physician can legally practice. These include obtaining the following:

- Employer identification number (EIN);
- State tax number;
- State medical license for every state in which the physician plans to practice;
- Drug Enforcement Administration (DEA) permit;
- Hospital privileges;
- Payer credentialing after receiving state license and DEA payment; and
- Medicare/Medicaid credentialing (855 form).

Plenty of time needs to be allowed for credentialing; some steps take several months. Many practices will not allow a new physician to begin employment until his or her residency is completed and all credentialing is complete.

Every physician must have a state license and a DEA permit to practice medicine. Also, most practices will not allow a new physician to begin work until the insurance carriers, such as Medicare and Medicaid, have credentialed the physician. After the physician has been credentialed, he or she can receive reimbursement for services rendered.

A physician's training license is not a state license. He or she must apply for licensure in every state in which he or she wishes to practice. For example, a group practice may have a satellite office in a neighboring state. In most cases, a state will allow the physician to practice there if he or she is licensed in a neighboring state and working for an organization with sites in both states, but this needs to be verified.

State medical license and DEA permit applications can each take three to four months to complete. Insurance carriers also take three to four months to process applications. Thus, each new physician can face a six- to nine-month process to get every credentialing obligation accomplished. All other credentialing requirements, including insurance panel credentials, flow from these two credentials.

To receive reimbursement for services rendered to patients, physicians must be credentialed with insurance carriers, including Medicare and Medicaid. Most practices will not allow a new physician to begin work until he or she has been credentialed by the insurance carrier(s). Also, most health insurance carriers require approval of hospital privileges before they will consider applications for provider participation, although some will process provider participation applications while hospital privileges are pending.

If an insurance carrier has not approved a physician for participation on its physician panel, it will not pay claims for his or her patients. New physicians who do not complete the credentialing process prior to seeing patients will cost the practice money.

Do not underestimate the time required for credentialing. The process can take up to nine months to complete, so the sooner the process is started, the sooner the physician can see patients and the practice can bill for services.

Obtaining Applications

- **Employer identification number.** Obtain an EIN from the Internal Revenue Service at www.irs.gov. Search the Web site with the phrase "employer identification number."

- **State license.** A state license is required for every state in which the physician plans to practice. Obtain the license from the state board of medical examiners, accessible via the Federation of State Medical Boards at www.fsmb.org. Many states also post this information online. A fee of several hundred dollars is to be expected to obtain a state medical license.

- **DEA permit.** Obtain this permit through the U.S. Department of Justice Drug Enforcement Administration. For telephone inquiries, call 800.882.9539, or visit the contacts page at www.usdoj.gov/dea/contactinfo.htm.

- **855 form.** This form from the Centers for Medicare and Medicaid Services allows the physician to bill for services provided to Medicare patients. Go to www.cms.hhs.gov for the application and information on how to complete it.

As with many medical practices, the practice administrator assists the physician in completing any required applications.

Chapter 6   # Monitoring the Peer Review Process[38]

IT HAS BEEN ARGUED that "...since lay people lack the ability to judge a physician's competence, the courts serve as a substitute for the marketplace in weeding out incompetent and careless doctors. There is no evidence to substantiate this argument. Lay judges and juries, and a courtroom battle between opposing medical experts, do not provide a substitute for objective peer review. ...Neither is there merit to the argument that damages for pain and suffering serve to punish "bad" doctors. Such payments for damages punish all policyholders, and in the final analysis it is the public who pays through higher health care fees, and in the case of government health care programs, through higher taxes."[39]

Every incident report, every patient complaint, and every request for medical record summary should trigger an investigation of the patient's medical record, and questionable situations should precipitate a peer review. A continuing problem with one physician can present a significant legal problem, especially if the physician is a partner in the group. Solid documentation of previous difficulties, the action taken, and the involved physician's response are required to prevent repercussions in the event the partners find it necessary to terminate a physician's services in the group. The partners should have the ability to buy out the offending physician's financial interest in the group should this become necessary.

Smaller groups (one to three physicians) present another problem. One physician cannot conduct a peer review on himself or herself; neither can one conduct a proper review on his or her partner. Even with three in the group, the one can claim the other two were "victimizing" him or her. These situations call for a reciprocal arrangement with other independent small group practices to ensure a total lack of bias.

If every physician will look on peer review as an effort for continuing improvement, rather than as questioning the physician's skills, the peer review process will work. After all, is not one of the goals of the physician to be the very best that he or she can be? Would s/he not welcome his or her peers pointing out an overlooked foible, rather than waiting for a lawyer and jury to point it out for him or her?

It is difficult to determine the impact of noncompliance with the standard or the cost/benefit ratio of the effort to initiate the standard. It must be remembered that not all costs of noncompliance are financial and neither are all the benefits of compliance. Even one medical malpractice claim, be it true or false, can be devastating to a physician, and his or her family.

▰ Employee Actions

Many doctors are aware of the important role played by their office staff in providing quality health care, but they may not realize that staff can also get them into malpractice trouble. Staff can also keep them out of trouble. "Lawsuits can occur because of your employee actions, or their failure to act, or simply because of their attitudes. Any employee who puts procedures before people in the name of practice efficiency is undermining the quality of care you provide, and that leads to patient dissatisfaction. And its disgruntled patients – angry for whatever reason – who are most apt to sue when there is a poor result."[40] Any efficient doctor knows that a quality, experienced, and competent nurse who can anticipate the doctor's orders is an immeasurable boon to his or her practice. "A pleasant, well mannered and competent nurse or secretary can make all the difference between having a satisfied patient or an angry, suit-prone one. The trick is to have the nurse stay within the limits of delegation. It is easy for them to fall into the trap of 'playing doctor.' When asked for a medical opinion the assistants' only appropriate answer is 'I don't know. The doctor will have to look at it.'"[41]

In a busy medical group office, the physician is vulnerable to employees not under his direct control. From the moment he walks in the door, the patient will be directed and channeled through a series of procedures, culminating finally in the examination room. If at any time the patient feels he or she has been mishandled, it is the physician, as well as the medical office as a whole, who will be blamed. Front desk personnel should be hired with specific talents in caring for people. They should have training in discerning emergency situations, erring, if necessary, on the cautious side. If it is necessary for a patient to wait because of delays, they should be informed plainly, given a chance to reschedule, and made as comfortable as possible should they decide to wait. Being told that the "doctor is running a few minutes behind" and then having to wait an hour to be seen results in a frustrated patient who is more inclined to initiate a claim should something go wrong. All too often, this situation is created by poor scheduling methods and/or physicians trying to see too many patients in a day.

Staff should understand that they must always tell the doctor when a patient complains. The doctor has a right to know when one of his or her patients is upset or annoyed with him or her or any part of the clinic. This may be the first indication of an impending claim. It is quite possible that a frank and caring conversation now may forestall more precipitous actions later. Besides, the patient is the "customer" and the reason for the staff-member's employment. They deserve adequate, if not special, attention.

A reliable method must be found to provide for front office staff to always relay messages and instructions in both directions. They should have well-designed message pads that convey all necessary information, including date and time of calls and messages, to the recipient, and they should be well trained in screening skills for telephone calls.

A possible innovation for a large office is a skilled message center to which patient calls are directed for screening and forwarding.

Pads of preprinted duplicate forms for referral bookings should be provided with a copy to the patient and one for the chart.

Peer Review Laws

Quality processes are governed by a variety of industry regulations and standards. In addition to the surveys provided by the Joint Commission on Accreditation of Healthcare Organizations (JCAHO), CMS and other accrediting and state agencies may monitor the health care organization for quality. The medical practice examiner should be knowledgeable about the specific organizations that conduct surveys and audits in the states where the practice has facilities. Whoever interfaces with regulatory agencies should remain apprised of changing regulatory information. This individual often seeks interpretation of regulation as it applies to the specific practices of the medical group, and distributes findings and works with the quality improvement process to facilitate change.

Peer review laws in many states protect quality records from discovery in an effort to ensure free communication about potential issues within the practice. Within that protection, peer review activity, credential files, and event reports are often considered protected information. In addition, many states have legislation and regulations that require reporting specified data elements for state monitoring. Some states are tracking specific disease categories; others may be monitoring treatment processes for specific diagnoses. Each state has its own specific laws regarding protection and reporting with which the medical practice executive involved in information management activities must be familiar.

Conclusion

This volume is dedicated to reviewing each task associated within the QualityManagement domain of the *Medical Practice Management Body of Knowledge*. The medical practice executive's role requires proficiency and aptitude in all four general competencies, and the knowledge and skills found inside the Quality Management domain (within the Critical Thinking Skills competency) are critical for the success of both the practice executive and the medical practice. By learning and mastering this domain, the practice executive will glean the skills required to effectively lead the organization toward success.

Exercises

THESE QUESTIONS have been retired from the ACMPE Essay Exam question bank. Because there are so many ways to handle various situations, there are no "right" answers, and thus, no answer key. Use these questions to help you practice responses in different scenarios.

1. A surgeon in your practice performed a medically necessary and successful surgery on a patient. Your practice is known for its excellent patient satisfaction and tries in every way to resolve issues to the patient's satisfaction. Your office staff failed to precertify the surgery, and the patient's insurance company refuses to pay the hospital bill. The patient, stating that your office assured her that they would handle the precertification, now insists that the practice should "take care of" the hospital bill or she will sue.

    What course of action would you take in this situation?

2. You are the administrator of a medical group. The nursing director approaches you for advice on how best to respond to a complaint from a nurse about a verbally abusive patient. This nurse refuses to care for this patient because he uses language she finds vulgar and offensive.

   Describe how you would handle this situation.

Notes

1. Reprinted from MGMA *Connexion*, July 2007, with permission of the Medical Group Management Association. All rights reserved.

2. D. Gans, J. Kralewski, T. Hammons, and B. Dowd. "Medical Groups' Adoption of Electronic Health Records and Information Systems," *Health Affairs* 24(5): 1323–1333.

3. Albert Barnett and Gloria Gilbert Mayer, *Ambulatory Care Management and Practice* (Gaithersburg, MD: Aspen Publishers, 1992), 291.

4. B. H. Bussell, "Managed Care," in R. Carroll (ed.), *The Risk Management Handbook for Healthcare Organizations* (San Francisco: Jossey-Bass, 2004), 517–520.

5. Ibid., 536.

6. C. Vincent, M. Young, and A. Phillips, "Why Do People Sue Doctors? A Study of Patient and Relatives Taking Legal Action," *Lancet* (1994) 343(8913): 1609–1613.

7. G. Amori, "Communication with Patients and Other Customers: The Ultimate Loss Control Tool," in R. Carroll (ed.), *The Risk Management Handbook for Healthcare Organizations* (San Francisco: Jossey-Bass, 2004), 821.

8. Anonymous.

9. S. K. Baker, *Managing Patient Expectations: The Art of Finding and Keeping Loyal Patients* (San Francisco: Jossey-Bass, 1999).

10. Institute for Healthcare Improvement, www.ihi.org/ihi.

11. W. Edwards Deming, *Out of the Crisis* (Cambridge, MA: Massachusetts Institute of Technology, Center for Advanced Engineering Studies, 1990), 166.

12. Amori, "Communication with Patients and Other Customers," 821.

13. Portions of this chapter were reprinted from *Benchmarking Success*, with permission from the Medical Group Management Association. All rights reserved.

14. R. Camp, "Benchmarking: The Search for Best Practices that Lead to Superior Performance, Part 1." *Quality Progress* (1989)22(1): 61.

15. D. Gans, "Benchmarking Successful Medical Groups to Improve Your Practice Performance." Presentation at MGMA Conference, Ohio, September 2006.

16. R. Camp, "Best Practice Benchmarking: The Path to Excellence." CMA Magazine (1998) 72(6): 10.

17. Ibid.

18. Camp, "Benchmarking," 61.

19. Ibid.

20. R. Camp, "A Bible for Benchmarking by Xerox." Financial Executive (1993) 9(4): 23.

21. Camp, "Benchmarking," 61.

22. Gans, "Benchmarking Successful Medical Groups."

23. Ibid.

24. Ibid.

25. Ibid.

26. D. Gans and G. Feltenberger, "Benchmarking Military Performance Using Civilian Metrics." Presentation at American College of Healthcare Executives Annual Conference, March 2007.

27. Wikipedia, "Baseline (configuration management)," http://en.wikipedia.org (2006).

28. M. Zairi and J. Whymark, "The Transfer of Best Practices: How to Build a Culture of Benchmarking and Continuous Learning, Part 2." *Benchmarking* (2000): 7(2): 146.

29. Gans and Feltenberger, "Benchmarking Military Performance."

30. Ibid.

31. Ibid.

32. National Committee for Quality Assurance, www.ncqa.org/ (accessed July 2005).

33. Kathryn Glass, *RVUs: Applications for Medical Practice Success* (Englewood, CO: Medical Group Management Association, 2003).

34. Medical Group Management Association, *Performance and Practices of Successful Medical Groups* (Englewood, CO: Medical Group Management Association, 2004).

35. Portions of this chapter were reprinted from *Physician Compensation Plans: State-of-the-Art Strategies,* with permission from Medical Group Management Association. All rights reserved.

36. "Clinical Pathways," www.openclinical.org/clinicalpathways.html (accessed Oct. 13, 2005).

37. The "Credentialing Process" portion of this chapter was reprinted from *Rx for Business Success: Joining a Medical Group Practice,* with permission from the Medical Group Management Association. All rights reserved.

38. A portion of this chapter was reprinted from the American College of Medical Practice Executives paper titled "Risk Management in the Medical Office" by Brian A. Baker, with permission from the Medical Group Management Association. All rights reserved.

39. M. Butler, *American Journal of Medical Genetics* (1990) 35(3): 319–332.

40. P. Milne, "Head injuries to pedal cyclists and the promotion of helmet use." *Accident and Analysis Prevention* (1988) 20(3): 177–185.

41. Ibid.

Index